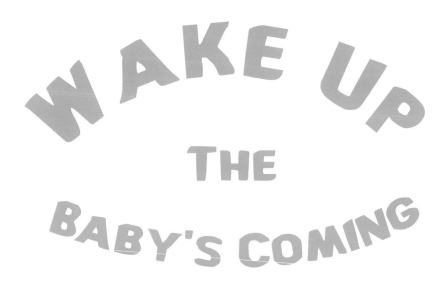

WAKE UP THE BABY'S COMING

BY
TIZIANA CICCONE

Strategic Book Publishing and Rights Co.

Strategic Book Publishing and Rights Co.
12620 FM 1960, Suite A4-507
Houston, TX 77065
www.sbpra.com

ISBN: 978-1-60860-685-6

To my children Daniel, Matthew and Liana
I am blessed to be your mother.

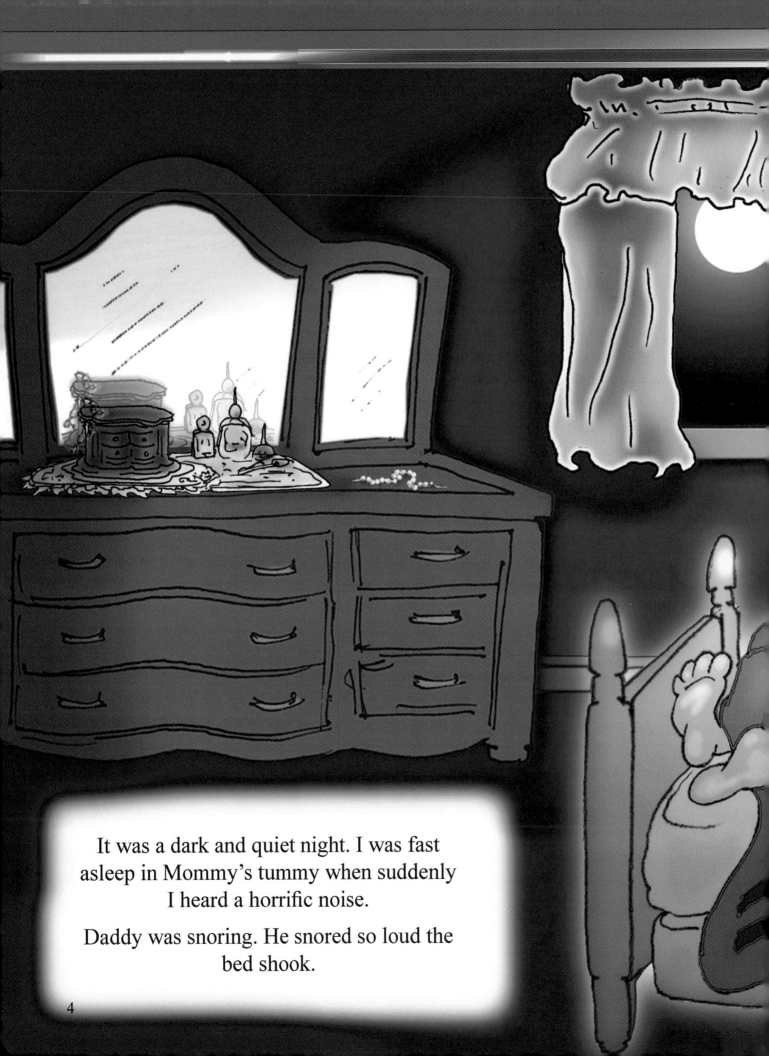

It was a dark and quiet night. I was fast asleep in Mommy's tummy when suddenly I heard a horrific noise.

Daddy was snoring. He snored so loud the bed shook.

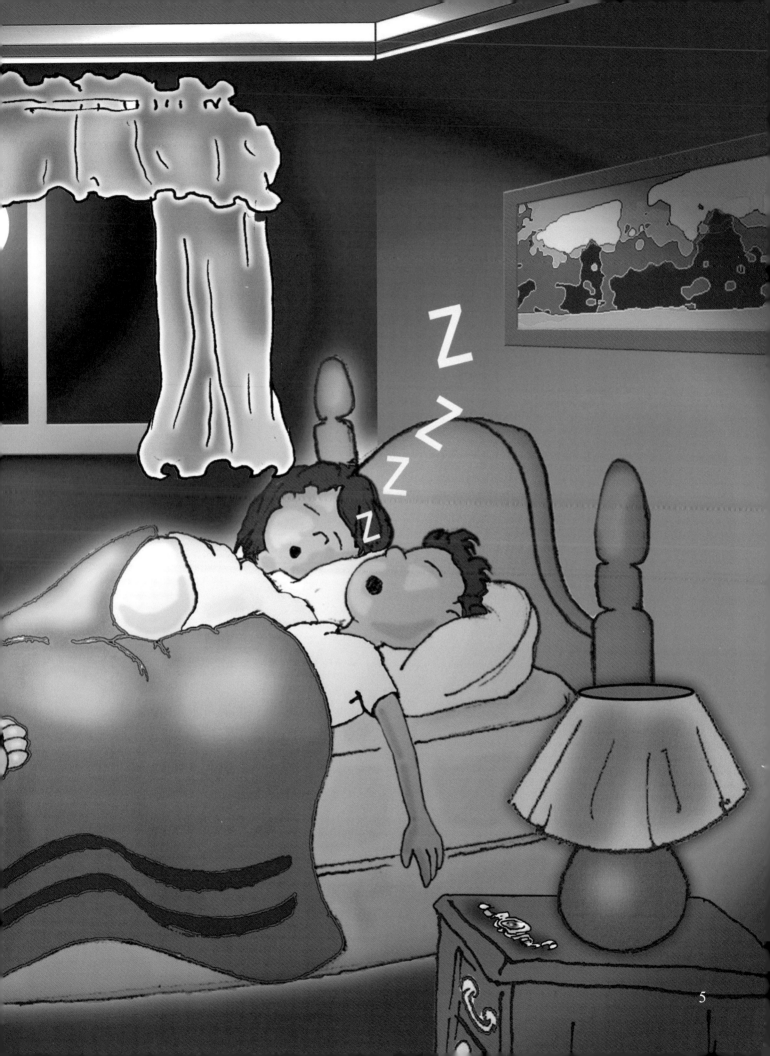

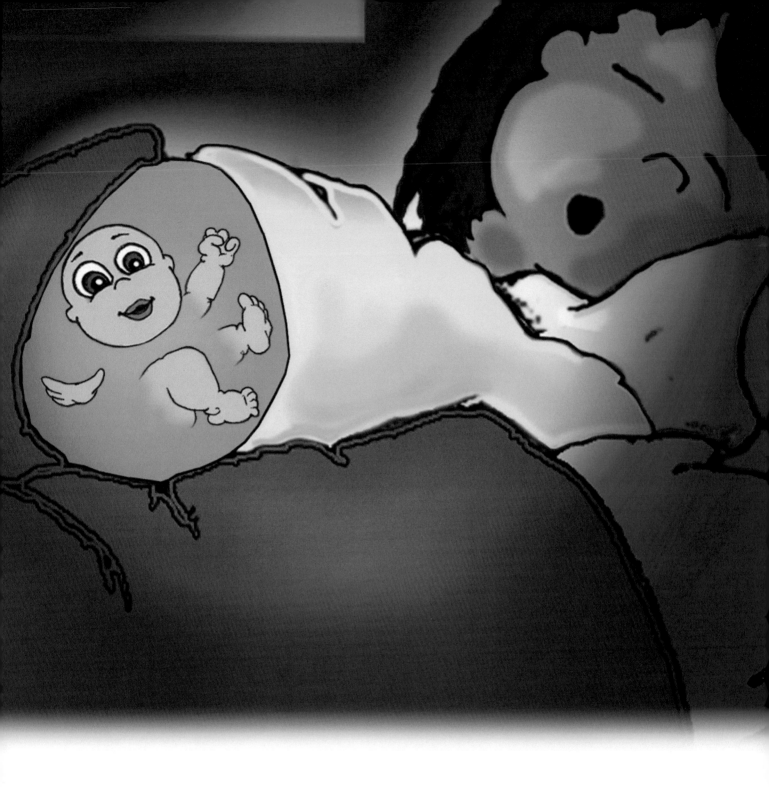

I wanted to go back to sleep, but he was making such a racket. I tried to move around in Mommy's tummy, but I was getting too big to fit. It was time for me to come out. I kicked Mommy three times to wake her up.

Whack, Whollop, Wham!

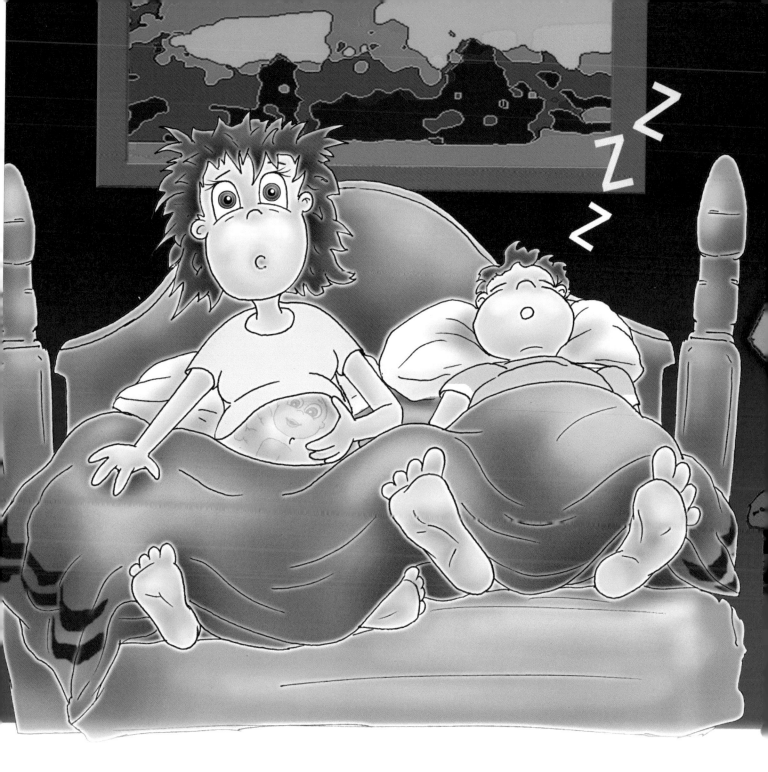

But she just stretched her arms, rubbed her tummy, and went back to sleep. So I kicked her harder.

Whack! Whollop! Wham!

Mommy woke up with such a startle.

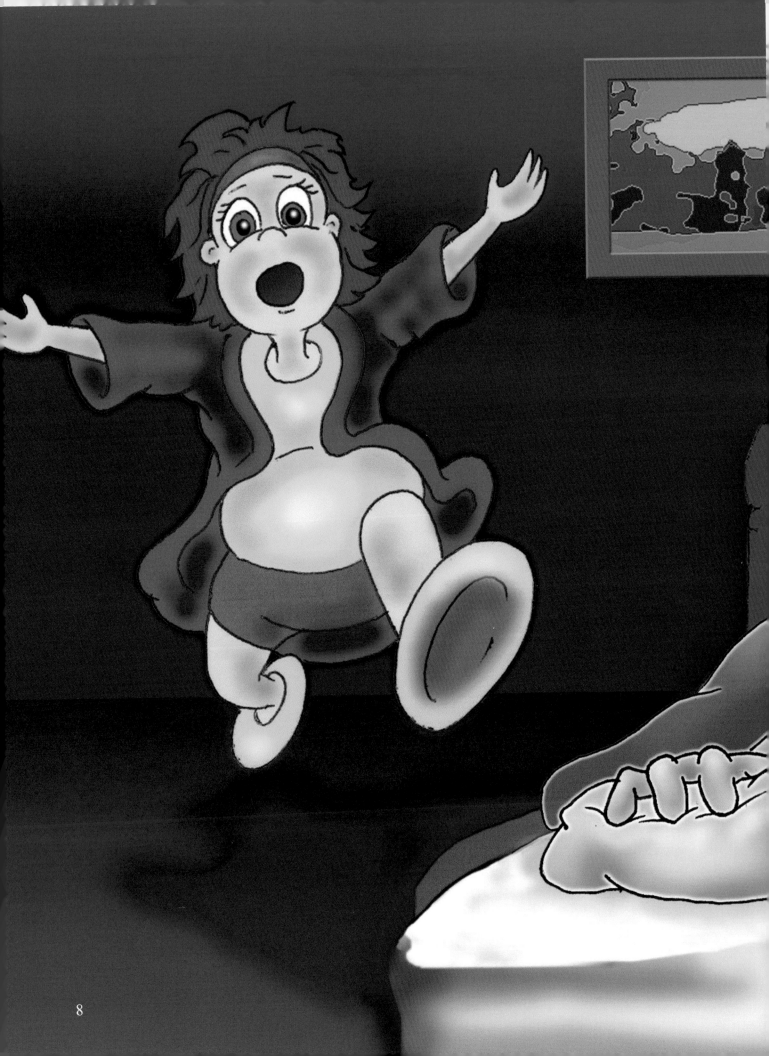

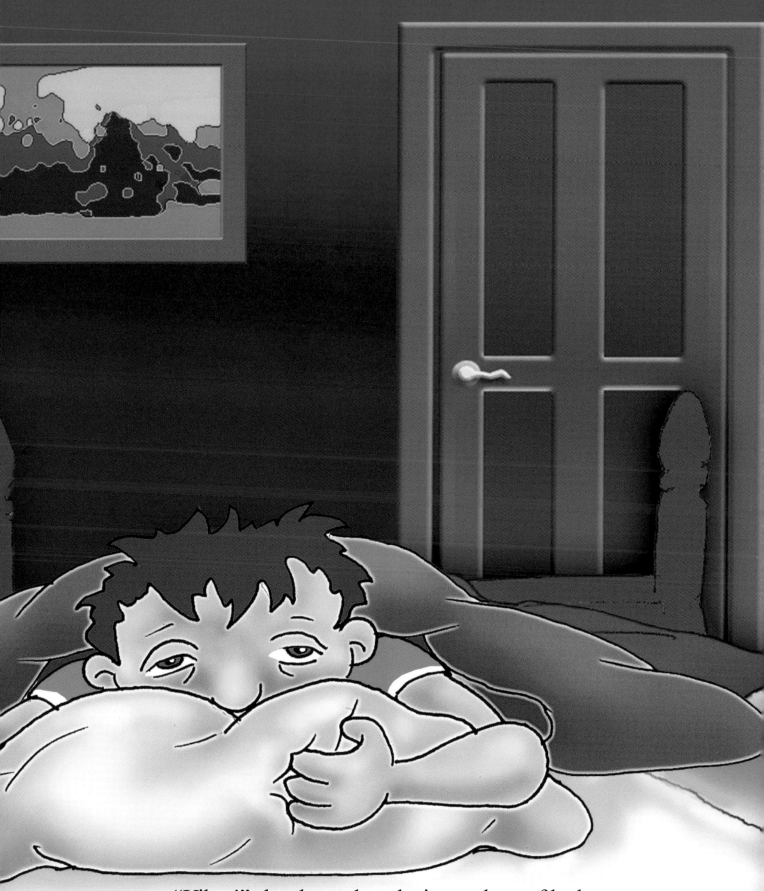

"Yikes!" she shouted as she jumped out of bed.

She looked at Daddy and ran around the room yelling, "Wake up! Wake up!
The baby's coming!"

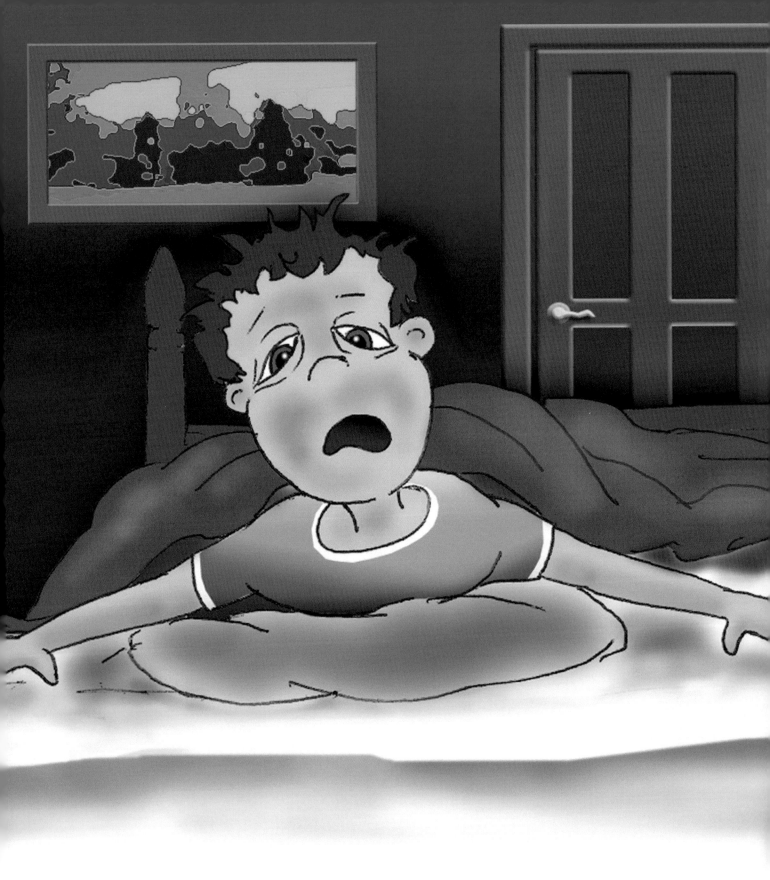

Daddy woke up all right!

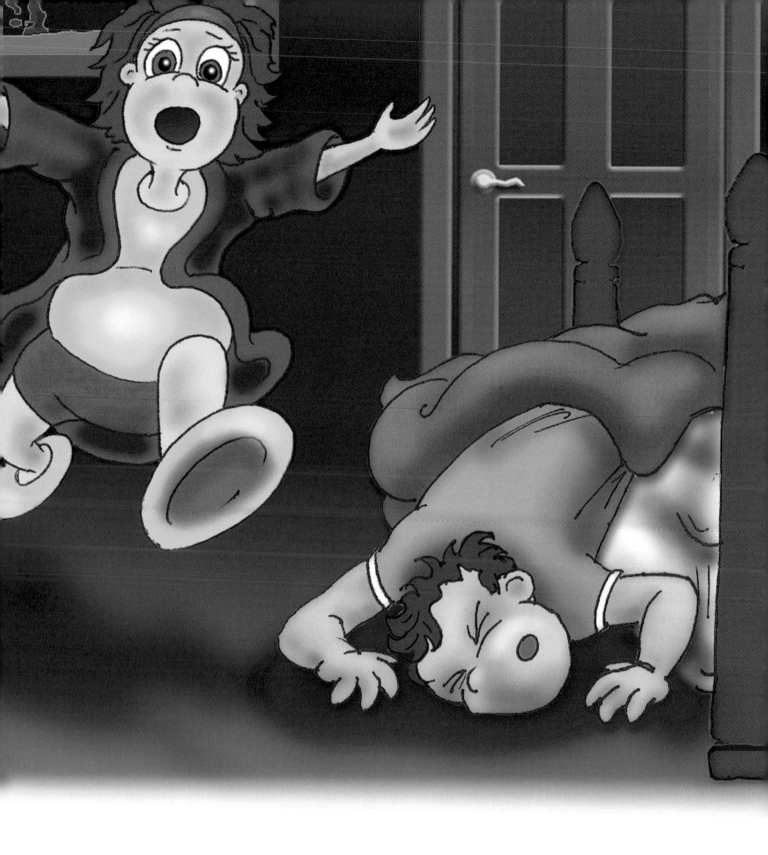

He rolled off the bed so fast he whacked his head on the floor.
"Oh no, is it really time to go?" he grumbled.

"It's time to go!" Mommy said.

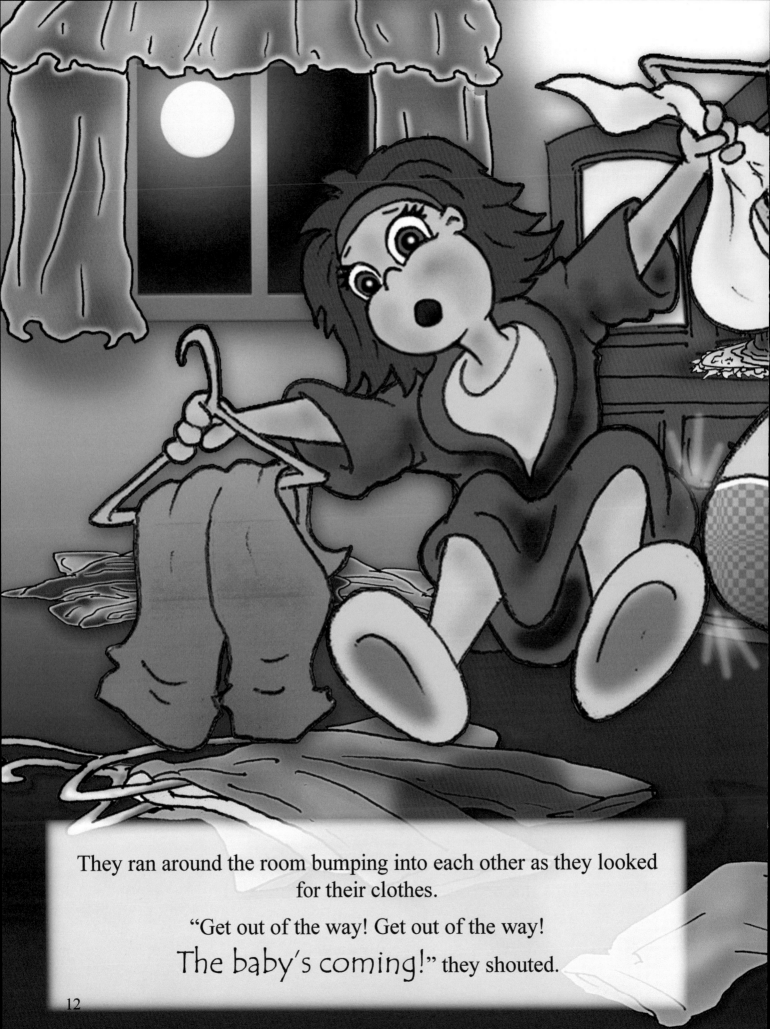

They ran around the room bumping into each other as they looked for their clothes.

"Get out of the way! Get out of the way! The baby's coming!" they shouted.

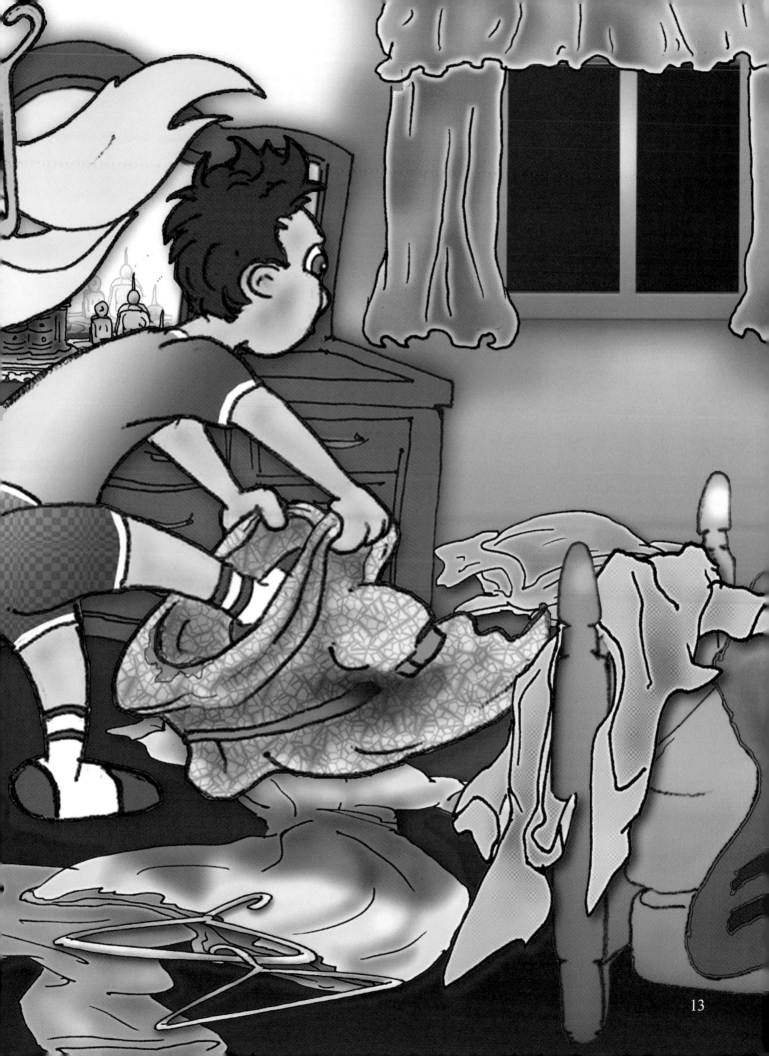

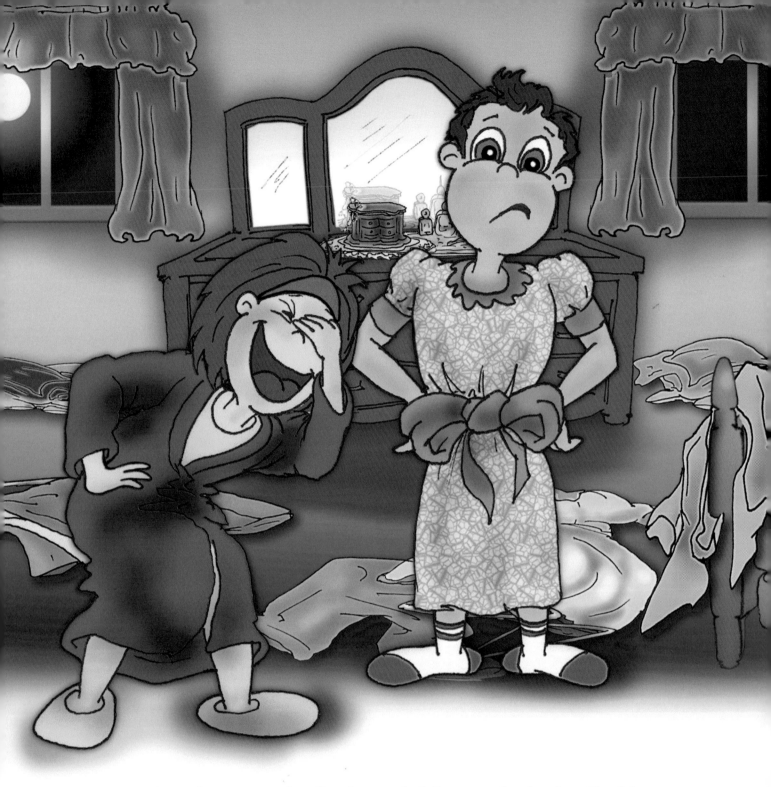

When they were finally dressed, Mommy looked at Daddy
and started to laugh.

He was wearing her dress.

Daddy didn't think it was very funny.

Mommy said, "Sorry, dear, but there's no time to change.
The baby's coming!"

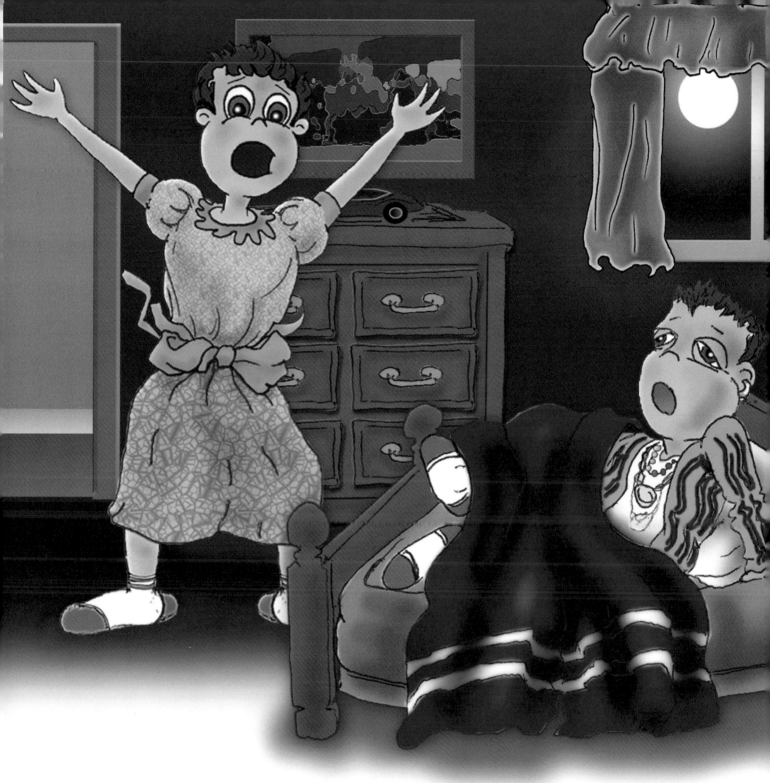

Daddy ran into my brother Matthew's room and yelled, "Wake up! Wake Up! The baby's coming!"

Matthew looked at Daddy and asked, "Why are you wearing a dress?"

"No time to explain. The baby's coming," answered Daddy.

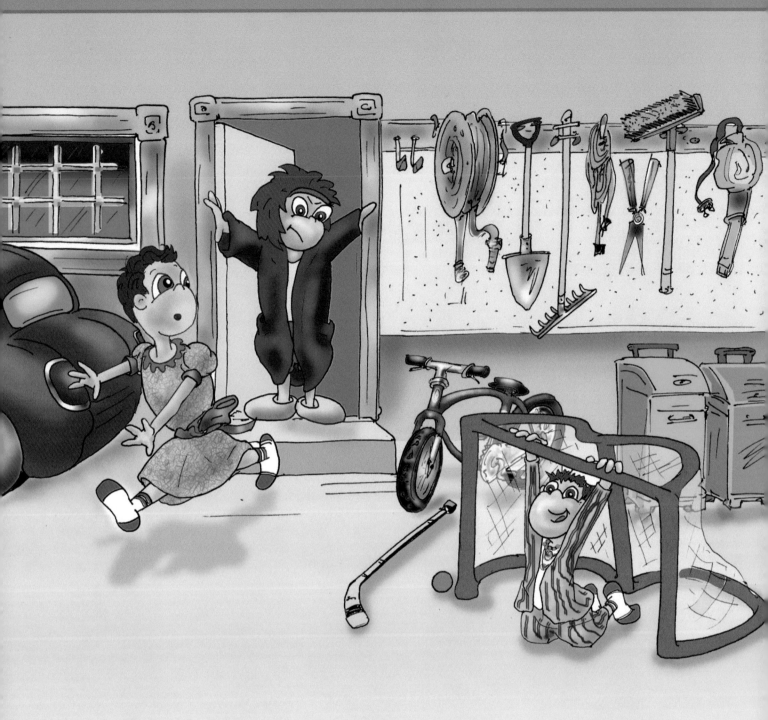

We hurried to the garage. Matthew wanted to play hockey
but Mommy said, "Not now! The baby's coming!"
So we jumped into the car.

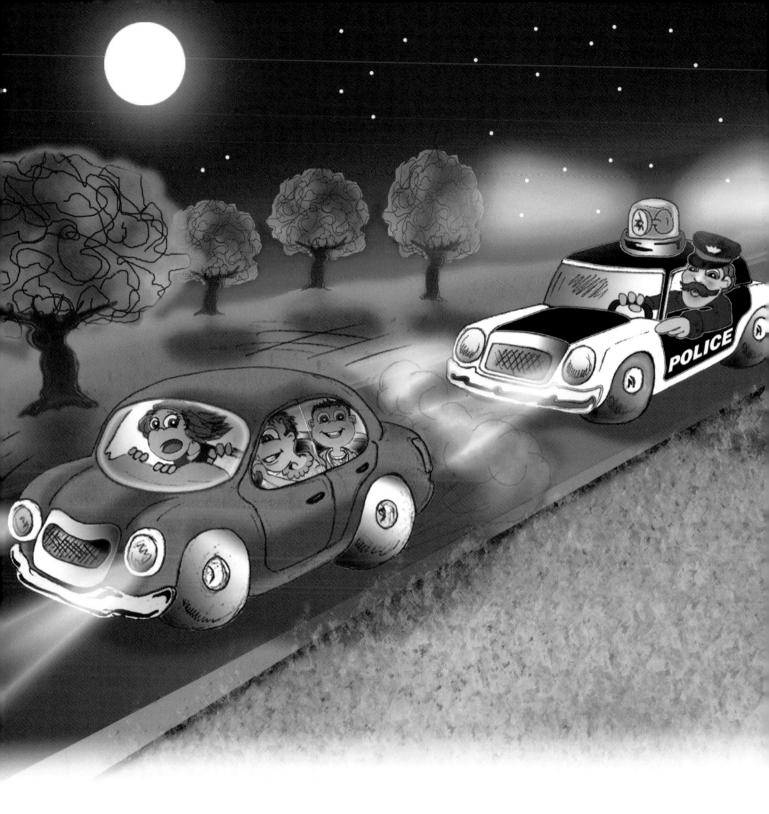

Off we went to the hospital.

A Ziggity Zag, a Zoom, and a Vroom went Daddy's car.
He was driving too fast. A police officer chased Daddy down the road.

The siren on his car went Woo! Woo! Woo!

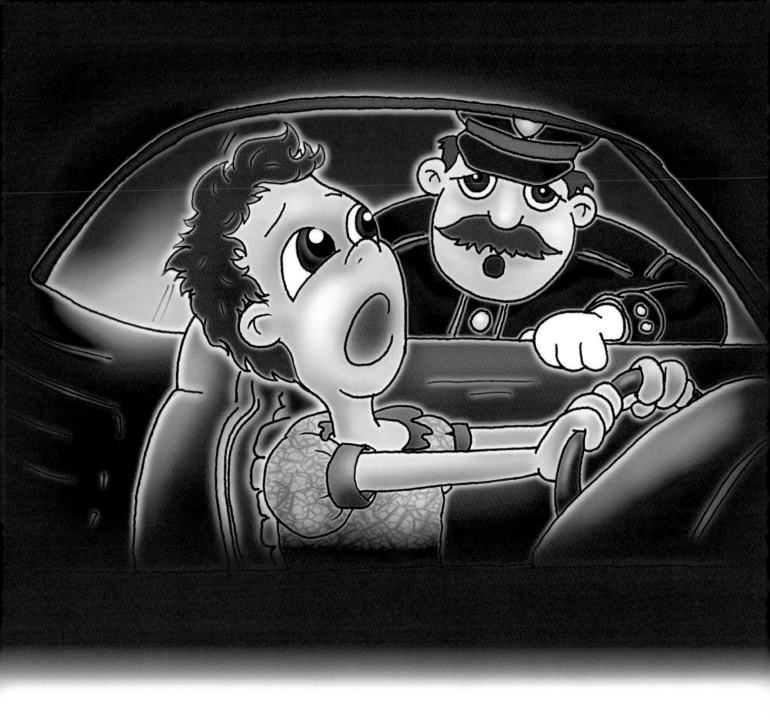

Daddy pulled over. The policeman stuck his head through the window. He looked at Daddy and said, "Excuse me, sir, but you're driving too fast and you're wearing a dress!"

My daddy said, "Sorry, Officer, but I have no time to explain. The baby's coming!"

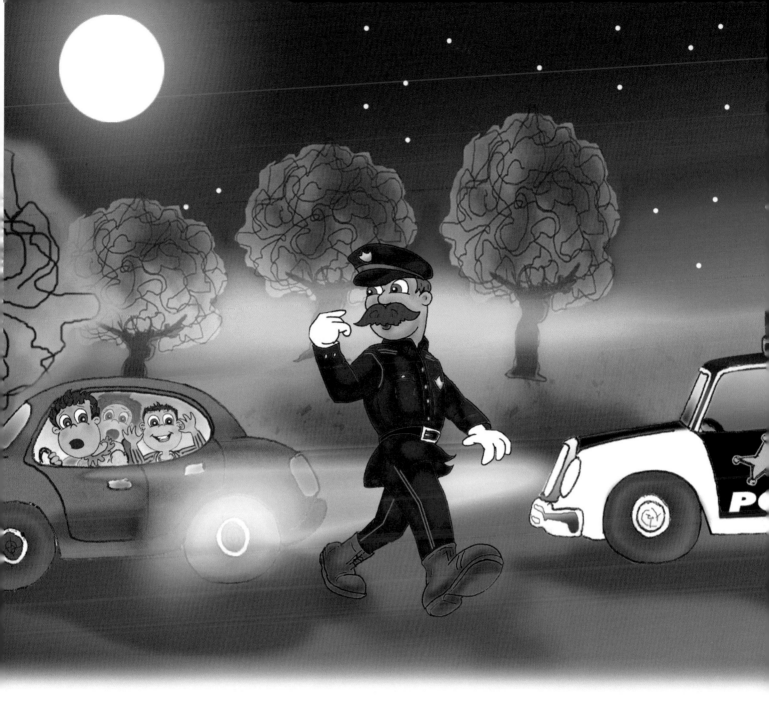

Oh no, follow me!" yelled the police officer.

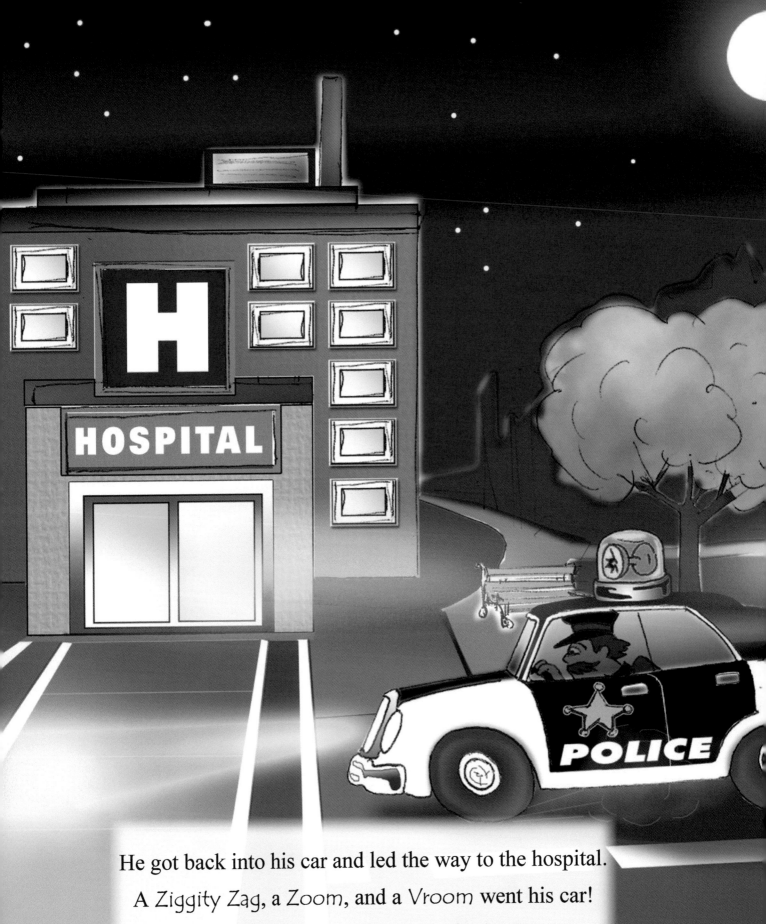

He got back into his car and led the way to the hospital.

A Ziggity Zag, a Zoom, and a Vroom went his car!

Now he was driving too fast!

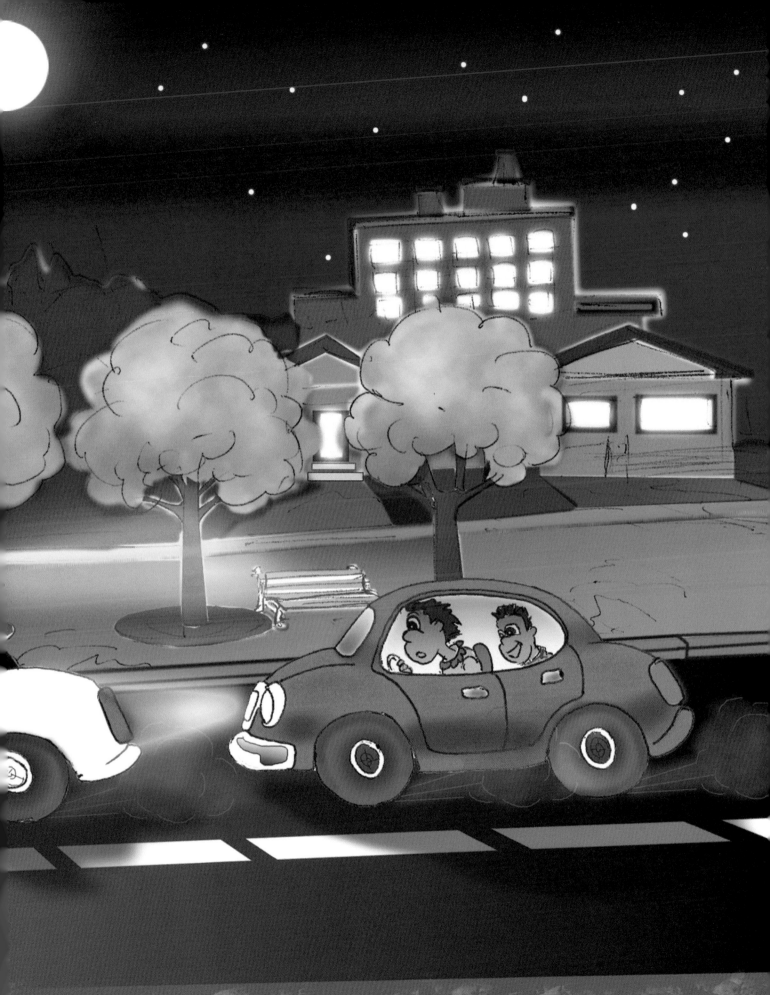

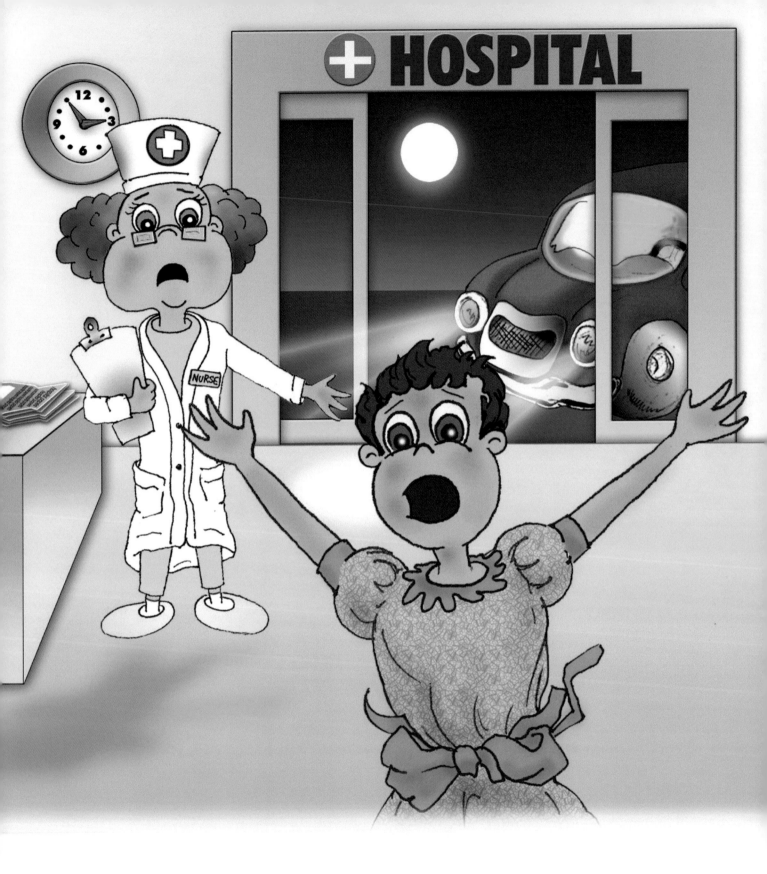

When we got to the hospital, Daddy ran into the emergency room and yelled,

"The baby's coming!"

The nurse looked at Daddy. "What baby?" she asked.

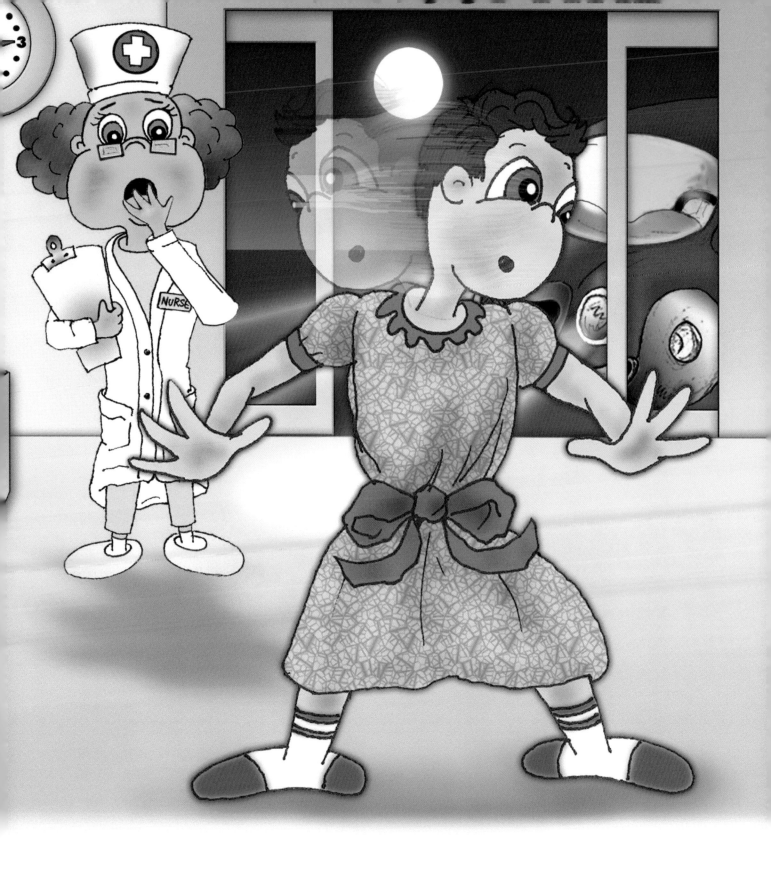

Daddy stopped and glanced around. "Oh no! I left them in the car!"

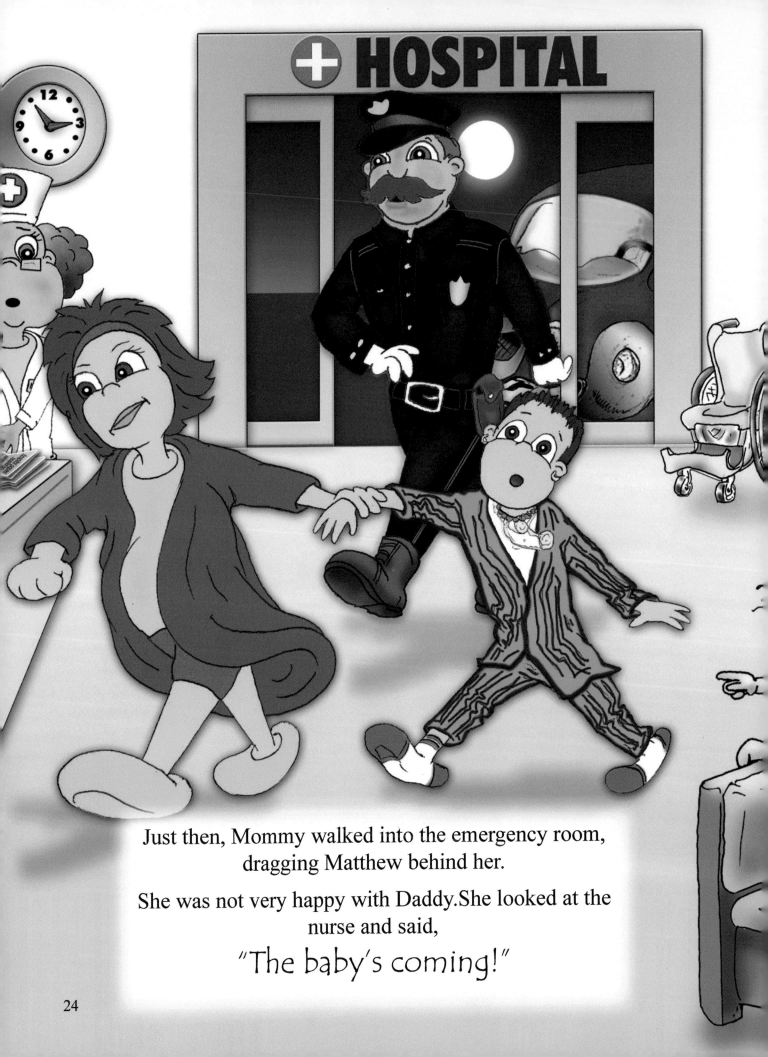

Just then, Mommy walked into the emergency room, dragging Matthew behind her.

She was not very happy with Daddy. She looked at the nurse and said,

"The baby's coming!"

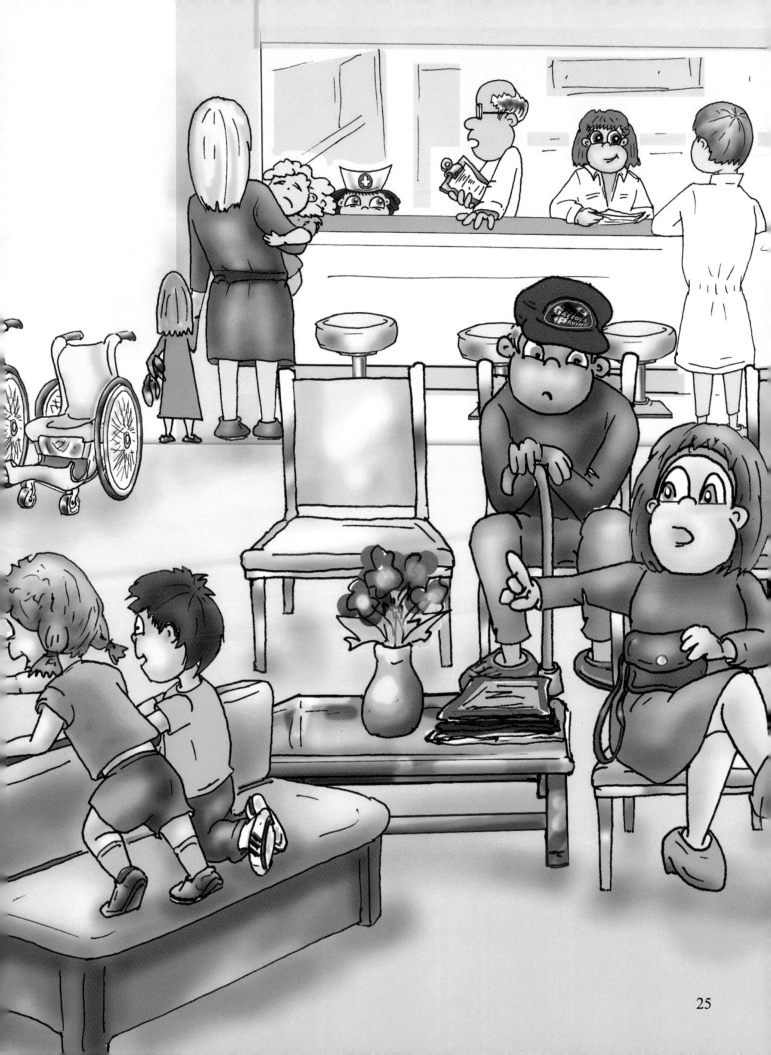

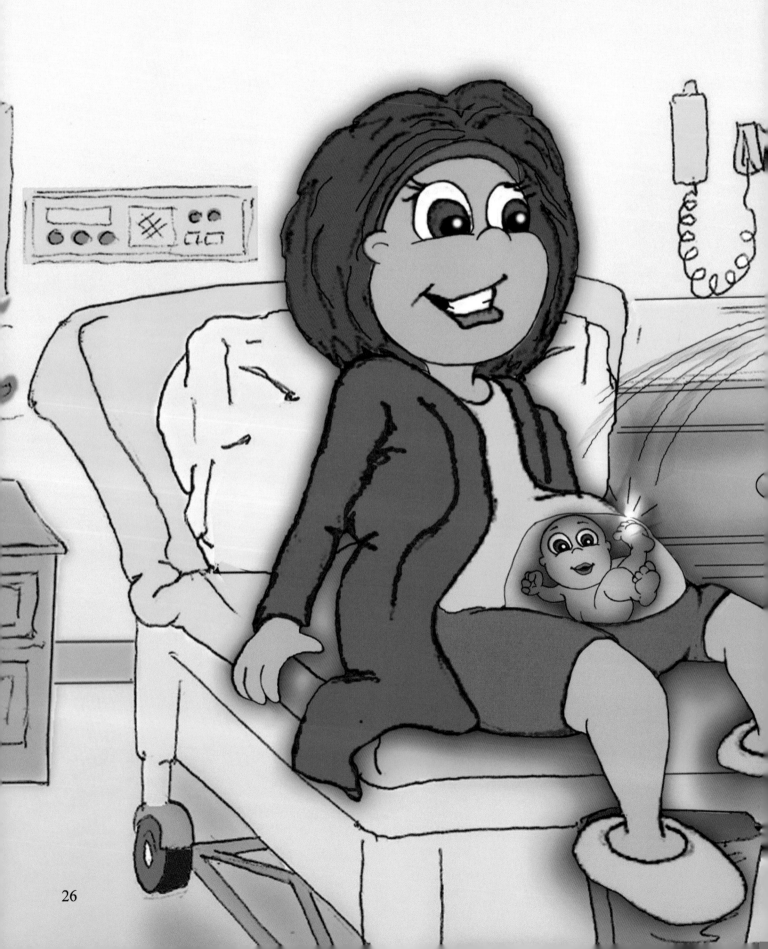

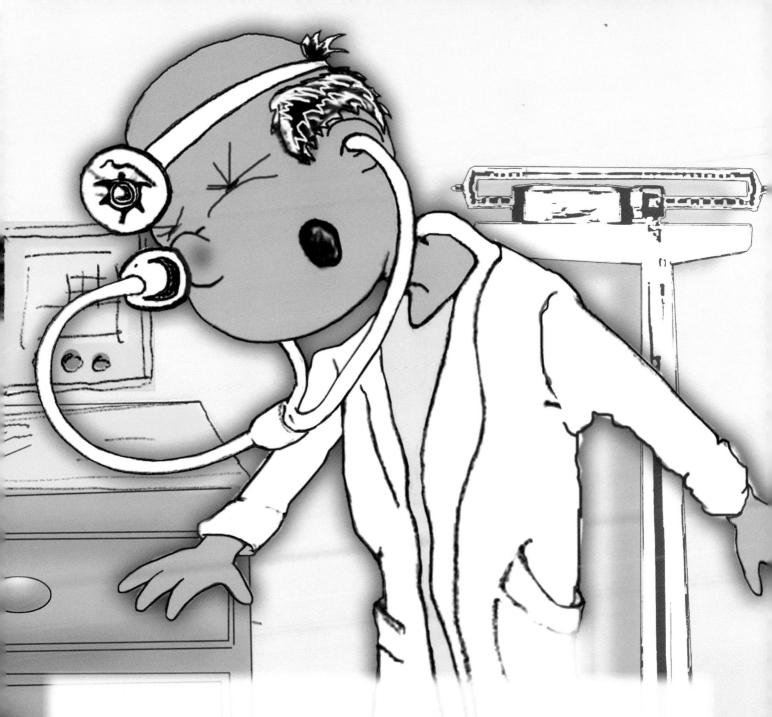

Mommy went into the examination room to see the doctor.
He checked her tummy with a stethoscope.
I kicked her three more times.

Whack! Whollop! Wham!

The stethoscope bounced off Mommy's tummy and
whacked the doctor in the nose.

Boink!

"Yes indeed, the baby is coming!" said the doctor.

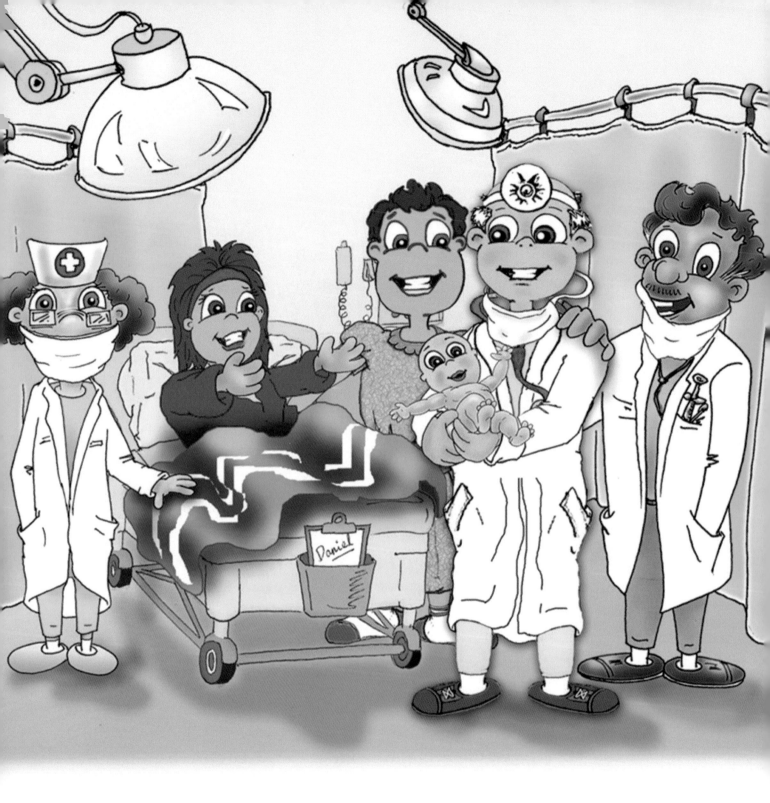

Then he took Mommy and Daddy to the delivery room where everyone
worked very hard to get me out.
When I was born the doctor said, "It's a boy!"

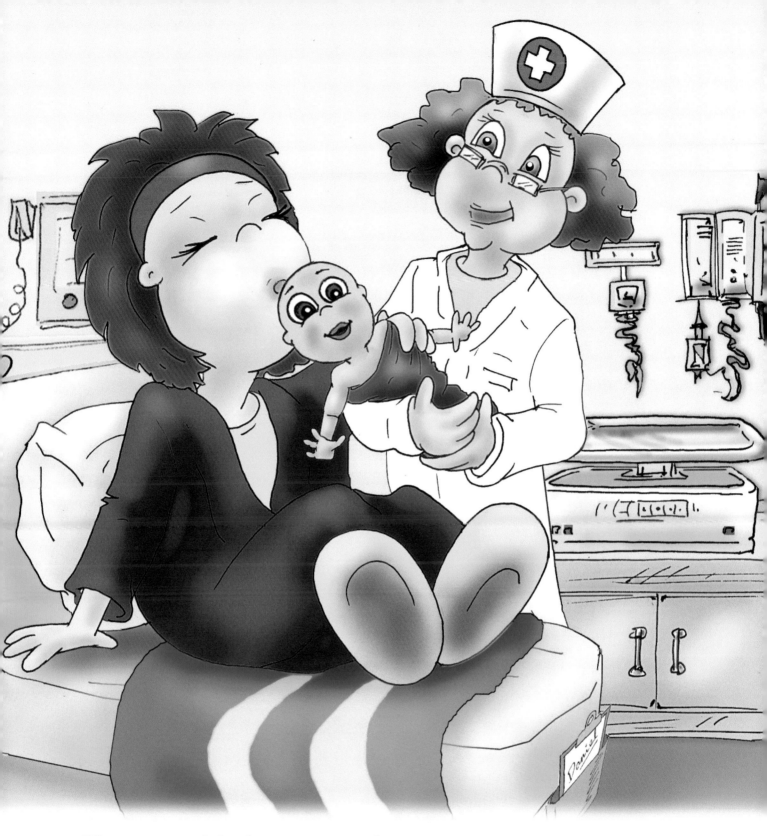

The nurse weighed me, measured me, and wrapped me in a blanket.
Mommy gave me a big kiss and said, "Welcome to our family, Daniel!"

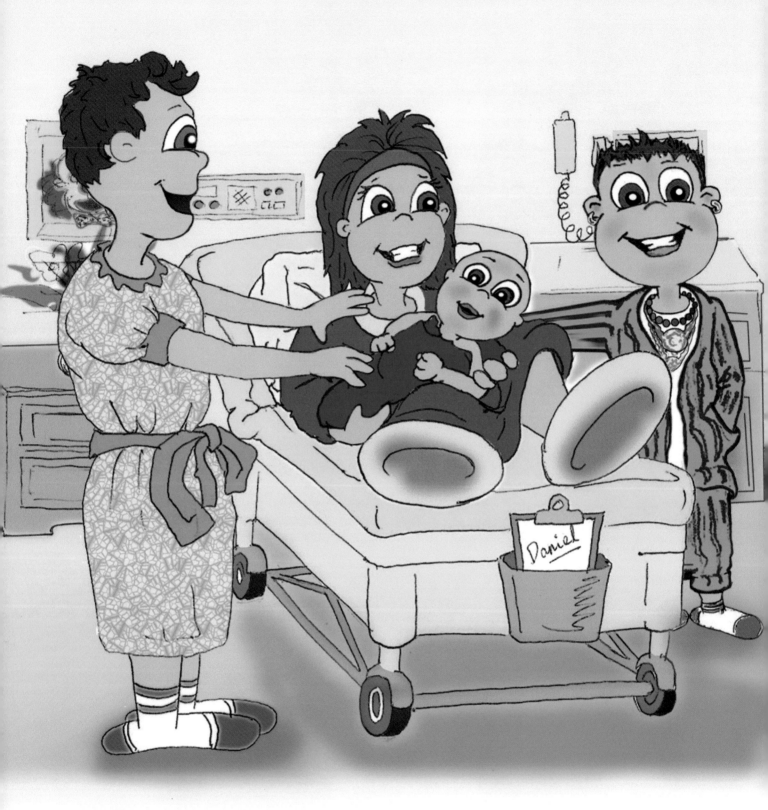

Matthew came into the room to meet me. He looked at my big head and tiny body and asked,"Is he human?"

Mommy and Daddy laughed.

I thought Matthew was silly.

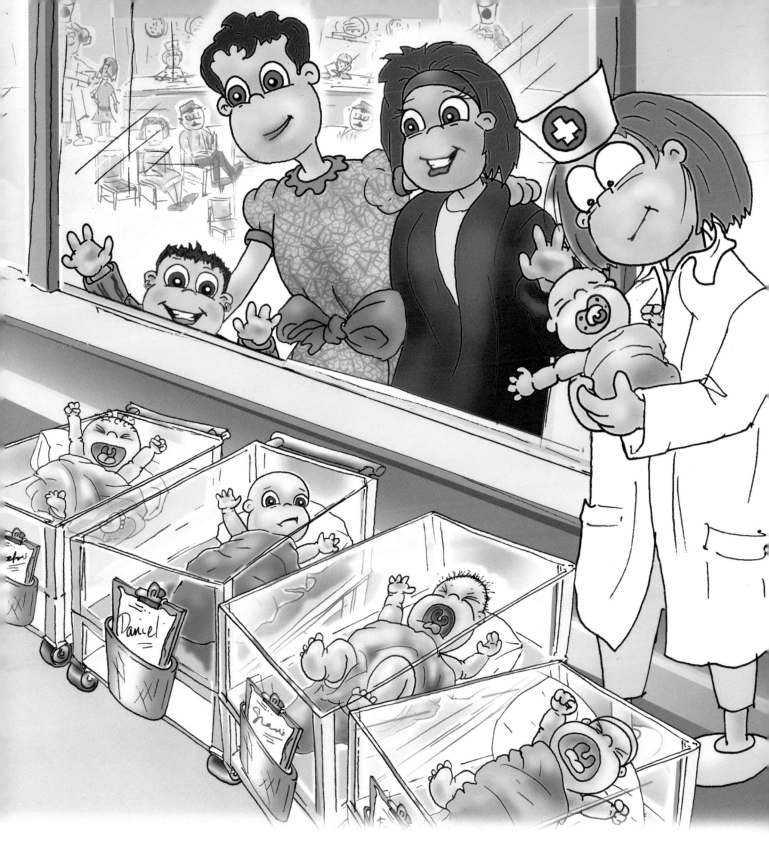

I spent the night in the nursery in an incubator because the doctor said I needed to stay warm. The other babies did a lot of crying, so it was hard for me to fall asleep.

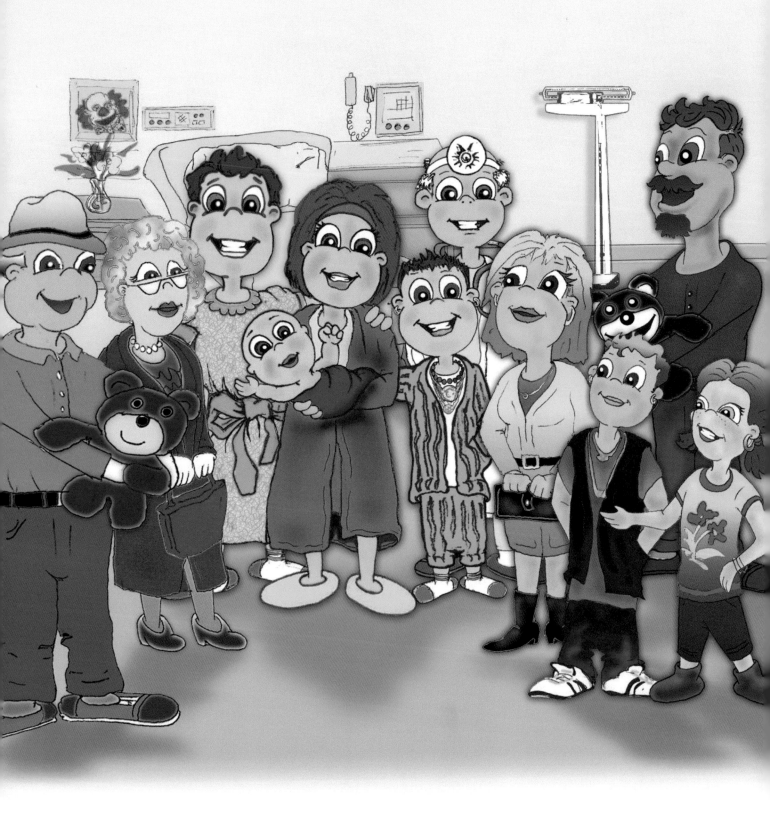

The next day my grandparents, aunt, uncle, and cousins came to visit me.

Everyone was happy because finally I was born!

CPSIA information can be obtained
at www.ICGtesting.com
Printed in the USA
LVIC01n1357041013
354781LV00004B

9 781608 606856